Contents

Foreword

There is a real buzz in the air: it's the sound of neuroscientists and teachers across the world talking to each other as they explore the potential of brain science to improve the experience of all learners. We felt that buzz first hand when we worked alongside groups of teachers in a recent research project, pooling our expertise from neuroscience and education, and sharing ideas about how to translate knowledge about the brain and learning into practical classroom advice.

We hope you will find the information in this Pocketbook exciting and that as you begin to use the tips and approaches described, you will start to recognise how having accurate knowledge about the brain can make for more effective teaching. Equally, by giving your pupils access to that same knowledge you can help them to become better learners.

Introduction

Why know about brain science?

Learning happens in the brain and what you as a teacher do affects the brains of the children you teach. Recent neuroscience research clearly demonstrates that the environment shapes and directly influences brain structure. This sort of research evidence is helping us to understand what underlying mechanisms may be at work in the interrelationship between the social situations we put learners in and how those learners develop.

What you do in the classroom is, over time, likely to affect the brain structure of the children you teach.

One field of study, sometimes known as **biological psychology**, is beginning to synthesise our understanding of the relationship between the social and the biochemical and has things to say that we believe are of great use to teachers. That's what this book is about.

Five reasons for buying this book

Some great reasons for finding out more about brain science and learning:

(1) Learning about the brain is fascinating and relevant; it makes for exciting professional development.

(2) Understanding the science of learning in the brain is a powerful way to inform teaching and have an impact on learning.

(3) There are many practical applications that can help teachers to improve their classroom practice.

(4) Research evidence shows that teaching children about how their brain learns can improve their motivation to learn and may in turn raise their attainment.

(5) It's fun!

What's covered and what's not

Every day new discoveries are being made in the field of brain science and we couldn't possibly hope to include everything there is to know in this Pocketbook. We also know, from working with many teachers and hundreds of children, that while some things are relevant and practically useful, others are not.

What's in

- The things that the teachers we have worked with tell us are useful
- Practical tips and ways to apply your learning in the classroom
- Easy-to-read explanations

What's not

- Everything there is to know about the subject
- Theoretical information that is just that
- Too much complex scientific terminology and labels

If, after reading this Pocketbook you want to find out more about the research into education and neuroscience, there's some suggested reading on page 125.

What is the brain for?

Your brain is a bit like a referee, trying to keep in check two opposing players: the thrill-seeker and the thinker.

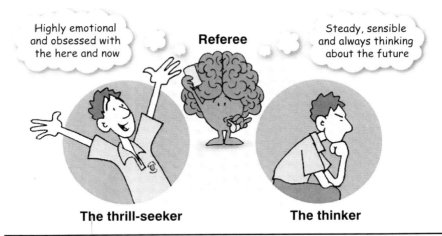

The thrill-seeker

The thinker

What is the brain for?

Of course, we don't actually have different personalities
inside us, but we do have incredibly sophisticated
machinery inside our skulls, machinery that has evolved
over millions of years to:

- Efficiently take in information
- Remember it for the future
- Weigh up the benefits of different courses of
  action: short-term satisfaction versus a greater
  gain in the long term

You'll see why children need special help with this
later in the book.

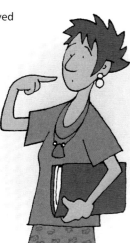

Nature or nurture?

How much of the improvement that learners make is down to you and how much is the result of genes?

- Brain connections that form automatically in early childhood as a result of genetic 'programming' contribute to only one third of intelligence
- It is environment and learned information that are critical in shaping brain structure, behaviour and intelligence
- Even identical twins, born with an identical blueprint to construct their brain, develop very different and unique personalities and traits

As a teacher, you are primarily responsible for shaping the connections inside your students' brains, connections that will remain in place for the rest of their lives. No other profession can make that claim.

You can do it!

Whereas some of the messages from psychology were occasionally perceived as being a little depressing from a teaching perspective (particularly things like IQ and notions of fixed intelligence), the latest brain science has some very positive messages about people's potential and the underlying basis for intelligence and ability. What we are now beginning to understand is this:

Much of what happens is not fixed by genetics or inheritance. Anyone can learn at any time in their life. Where learning is concerned – **You can do it**. However, you may need to change your current way of doing things to adopt methods that promote better retention and memory.

This is a challenge for all teachers because it emphasises further what we know from education research; namely that the quality of learning cannot be better than the quality of your teaching.

What to tell your learners about this

We know from research carried out by the Institute for the Future of the Mind (Oxford University/CfBT Education Trust) that when your learners know about the brain and about how learning and memory works, it has an effect on their **attitudes** to learning which in turn has the potential to raise **attainment**.

As well as sharing some of the key knowledge in this book with your pupils, it is particularly important that they understand three key points:

1 The brain is 'plastic'. It constantly grows and changes in response to the environment and what you experience. This is known by neuroscientists as **plasticity**.

2 No two brains are the same.

3 The brain grows and develops during a whole lifetime.

This challenges the notion of fixed intelligence. It points to the potential of everyone to achieve more, whatever their age, and to the importance of catering flexibly for individual differences in learning situations.

A summary of brain bits

The brain bits labelled on the next two pages play a leading role in learning and you will encounter them throughout this book.

First, you will want to familiarise yourself with the four **lobes** and the things that they are largely responsible for.

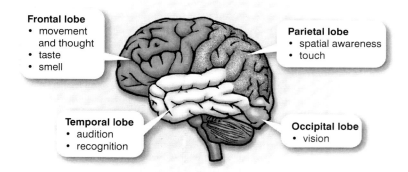

Frontal lobe
- movement and thought
- taste
- smell

Parietal lobe
- spatial awareness
- touch

Temporal lobe
- audition
- recognition

Occipital lobe
- vision

A summary of brain bits

If we cut the brain in half down the middle you can see some of its inner structure.

There's more about the structures that evolved and how we are defining them on pages 21 and 22 where we talk about the idea of there being three brains:

- The **hindbrain** (the really old bit)
- The **midbrain** and **limbic system**
- The **forebrain** (the wrinkly outer layer)

However, it's important to remember that the whole brain is active the whole time, as we'll discuss later.

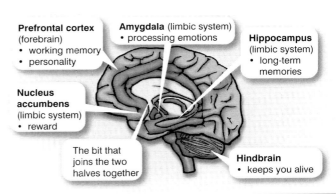

Prefrontal cortex (forebrain)
- working memory
- personality

Amygdala (limbic system)
- processing emotions

Hippocampus (limbic system)
- long-term memories

Nucleus accumbens (limbic system)
- reward

The bit that joins the two halves together

Hindbrain
- keeps you alive

What scares a neuroscientist?

Brain science has a lot to offer you and your classroom, but there are limits to how it can help. The limits relate to what neuroscientists do and what they don't do.

- Neuroscientists DO look at the brain in lots of different ways, starting at a very low level; for example, some will look at individual genes
- Neuroscientists DON'T tend to work closely with children or study normal behaviour in a group environment

As teachers, you do what neuroscientists don't, and it's important to understand that conclusions drawn at the level of individual genes, for instance, are unlikely to have any direct relevance in your classroom. Therefore, teachers and educators need to be cautious in using findings from research that is far removed from the classroom.

What's in the rest of the book

The next two sections will give you a basic understanding of brain structure and some key understanding about the brain and learning from a neuroscience perspective. We include some ideas for teaching children about the brain and learning and suggest strategies to support learning in the classroom.

We then look in detail at what we know about the neuroscience of memory and follow up with a series of practical teaching tips and strategies before looking at brain development and some controversial questions that arise as a result of how neuroscience is challenging our thinking.

We end with a reflective summary of the key learning in the book, suggestions for what you might do next and a further reading section.

Planning your learning journey

You may now like to take a moment to reflect on what you want to get out of this Pocketbook.

- You may be interested in simply improving your knowledge of the brain so that you are more up-to-date. In which case you will be particularly interested in the early sections and the 'future issues' section starting on page 113

- If you want to know more about what brain science can tell you about building on your existing good practice, you may want to pay particular attention to the middle sections

- If you want to find out more about specific learning difficulties or learning disabilities such as ADHD and dyslexia, this is covered on pages 99 to 103

- If you want to know how you can teach your learners about the brain, there are some fun activities and suggestions in the following sections

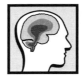

Brain Bits

What's in this section and why

Eeeuuggh, it's disgusting

Wow, that's amazing!

What's that wrinkly bit at the back for – the bit that looks like a cauliflower?

These are all comments shouted out by schoolchildren (and teachers!) as they handled real human brains at one of the regular outreach events we deliver.

Teachers tell us that they (and their students) have learned three things from the sessions:

1. Basic information about the brain is easy and fun to learn.
2. Knowing how the brain is wired together can help you better understand what it can and can't do.
3. Learning some simple brain facts can change how you view the limits of your own ability – for the better.

This section covers how the brain allows us to do all that we can, what the different parts of the brain are for and how you can use this information in the classroom.

Oh yes, the sessions also taught us never to show children real brains just after lunch!

Three for the price of one

Thinking of the brain in three parts can help you to understand it:

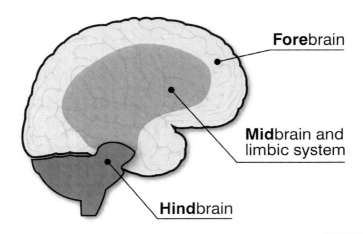

Forebrain

Midbrain and limbic system

Hindbrain

What the three parts of the brain do

Hindbrain – evolved first and is shared with animals as simple as reptiles, which is why it's sometimes called the **reptilian brain**. Though it's important, it's mostly concerned with just keeping you alive! It doesn't do anything as fancy as the bits higher up.

Midbrain and Limbic System – if you've ever wondered why it's so difficult to resist that piece of chocolate cake, look no further. Blame your midbrain; it gives you your basic drives.

Forebrain – consists of the most recently evolved structures in the brain (the cortex). It's your forebrain that enables you to use reason and logic to solve complex problems, plan for the future and perceive the world so sensitively and clearly.

The next few pages explain why we need each brain area and why this information is important in the classroom. You will also learn how you can excite different brain areas when teaching.

Staying alive!

What you need to know about the **hindbrain**:

- Some animals only have a hindbrain, which doesn't make them terribly clever
- The hindbrain is only worried about staying alive, and not about learning algebra!
- Although you have much more than just a hindbrain sitting inside your skull, it can still play a big – and largely negative – role in learning. Danger causes the hindbrain to spring into action to get you to fight or flee (reducing the influence of other areas of the brain that allow for thought, reason and higher order learning)

Maintaining a positive emotional climate in the classroom by controlling your own emotions as a teacher (and using a bit of humour!) is a great way to keep the children's hindbrains in check and keep them happy while you deliver the information that their **forebrains** need to develop more interconnectivity. (There's information about stress and learning on page 50.)

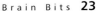

Gimme, gimme, gimme

What drives behaviour? Why do learners sometimes find it so difficult to concentrate on studying when it's nice and sunny outside? Why does chocolate cake always look so appealing? Scientists are still grappling with these questions but now know enough to pinpoint a group of brain structures – collectively known here as the midbrain and limbic system – that causes behaviour to 'lean' in certain directions.

- Much of behaviour, and even thought, is directed by unconscious emotions that have their origins in your midbrain and limbic system
- They 'push' you towards things that give you pleasure, and 'pull' you away from things that have previously made you anxious or afraid – and you're often totally unaware of this!

Negative emotions are particularly powerful because the connections between these emotions and the events that produce them are particularly strong and can last a very long time. (There's more about emotions and learning later in the book.)

Basic instincts

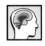

Neuroscientists love pointing to brain structures and telling you what they do. But how could knowing about the **hindbrain** and **midbrain** help you in the classroom?

Together, they are known as the **brainstem**. Think about the following scenario and what kind of reaction the brainstem might have:

Without warning, you announce one day that your pupils will take an exam immediately that will determine their Maths set for the next year.

Their brainstems will go wild after hearing this, and you don't want your learners controlled by their panicky brainstems! To ensure that the brainstem isn't interfering with their thoughts and actions, make sure your students have sufficient support and preparation before 'anxious events' such as exams to help other, more sensible parts of the brain calm the brainstem. Also, have fun when revising – avoid making it scary.

Hello? Is there anybody in there?

If neuroscientists had to point to a part of the brain that was responsible for making you you (the part that makes you the life and soul of the party or somebody more introverted; or that determines whether you enjoy or hate gambling and how morally-minded you are) they would point to your **forebrain**. In particular, they would point to the front of your forebrain: your **frontal lobes** (which include the **prefrontal cortex**). (See diagrams on pages 14 and 5.)

However, the frontal lobes are only as effective as the information that they are provided with. This is why the quality of your subject knowledge as a teacher is so important. It is also why, however much we learn about the brain from a biological and psychological perspective, the skills of a teacher will always be the determining factor in a child achieving his or her potential.

The big 'but' of brain structure

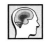

Although the idea of distinct brain divisions is a useful way of talking about the brain, and it is true that the sections look very different and have different functions, the truth is the whole brain works together all the time and in all activities. It's a bit like an orchestra with all instruments playing at once, then one or more instruments play a little louder.

There's nothing wrong with teaching children to recognise different ways that they are able to learn **but** quite another thing to say that these have something to do with very specific brain structures.

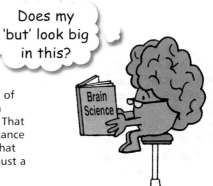

Does my 'but' look big in this?

Because what you do as a teacher reaches all parts of the brain all the time, you are constantly walking a tight rope to determine which area takes the lead. That takes us back to our earlier point about the importance or emotional climate, as some parts of the brain (that you really don't want to take the lead) are always just a small step away from increased activation.

Fun ways to teach this – plasticine brains

There are lots of fun ways to teach your pupils about the three main divisions of the brain. A very simple idea is to get them to make brains out of plasticine using a different colour for each division. Once they have done this, ask them to make a brain for different situations, where the biggest part would show which bit of the brain is in charge! Here are a few examples:

- If you suddenly spotted a grizzly bear in front of you (**hindbrain**)
- When you are eating a large piece of chocolate cake (**midbrain and limbic system**)
- When you are doing your homework (**forebrain**)

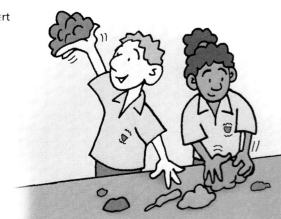

Fun ways to teach this – mythical creatures

Once you have shown your students that the brain is made up of the **hindbrain**, **midbrain and limbic system** and **forebrain**, you can teach them about the different **lobes** of the forebrain. An excellent way to do this is with the mythical animal game!

For each student you will need either four colours of plasticine or two sets – one large, one small – of cardboard cut-outs of the four different lobes: **frontal**, **parietal**, **occipital** and **temporal** (see page 14).

Ask your students to put together four lobes to make up the brains of mythical creatures. For example a cross between a bat and eagle might have excellent hearing from the bat and excellent vision from the eagle giving them big temporal and occipital lobes.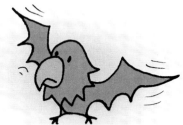

Fun ways to teach this – become Pinocchio

Though your brain is incredibly clever, it is only as good as the information you feed it. If you don't feed it the right information, it will attempt to fill in the blanks itself and have a guess at what it thinks is going on! Hmm... ever had that happen in the classroom when you haven't explained something well? You can demonstrate how it works with 'The Pinocchio Illusion':

1. Find two chairs and place one in front of the other.

2. Find a (good) friend and ask them to sit on the chair in front.

3. Sit on the chair behind, close your eyes and reach round with your dominant hand to tap and stroke your friend's nose.

4. At the same time, use your non-dominant hand to simultaneously tap and stroke your own nose.

5. If you do this for at least 30-60 seconds you may start to feel like your own nose is several feet in front of you! Like most experiments, this won't work with everyone but most people will find an effect.

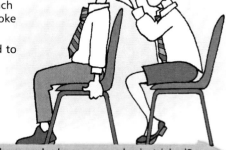

So how and why was your brain tricked?

What just happened?

The Pinocchio illusion should have made you believe that you had a nose that was incredibly long. The sensation of your nose being tapped at precisely the same time as you were tapping your friend's nose confused your brain into thinking that your friend's nose was actually your nose! Your eyes being closed meant your brain couldn't correct such a bizarre idea.

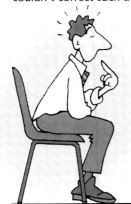

This goes to show that your brain's perceptual skills aren't perfect and, unless it receives the right kind of information, it can even be tricked into thinking your body parts are moving around.

A fun variation on the above that works even better is to get a third person to tap your nose instead, at exactly the same time that you tap the nose of the friend sitting in front of you.

Think, feel, do

Being **self-aware** has given us a huge evolutionary advantage – not only are we able to think, we are also able to think about our thinking! This means that we have the ability to control and manage the more primitive part of the brain (what people like Daniel Goleman* call 'emotional intelligence') and as neuroscientist Antonio Damasio**, has pointed out, all action and thinking is underpinned by emotion.

1. Get your class to write the words 'Thinking', 'Emotions' and 'Actions' on three pieces of paper and place them in a triangle on the floor.

2. Ask them to think about a time when they got everything wrong in terms of relationships.

3. Have the pupils stand on each of the spaces in turn and think about what was going on in each of the areas.

4. Ask them: Which area was dominating too much? Which one did they need to use more? Asking these sorts of questions often helps children to identify things in their attitude and behaviour that they were unaware of.

5. Get them to think about what they would do differently next time.

*_Emotional Intelligence: why it can matter more than IQ_ by Daniel Goleman, Bloomsbury (1995)
**_The feeling of what happens: body and emotion in the making of consciousness_ by Antonio Damasio, Vintage (2000)

Introduction

 Brain Bits

 The Learning Process

 The Neuroscience of Memory

 In the Classroom

 The Developing Brain

 Future Issues for Brain Science in the Classroom

 Reflective Summary

The Learning Process

What's this bit going to give you?

Although neuroscience can't help you to understand the social process level of learning in the same way as other research methods that are more qualitative or observational, it can, nonetheless, help teachers to understand some of the underlying processes. This section covers:

- Those areas of neuroscience that teachers tell us are helpful in supporting them to develop their pedagogy (particularly in relation to retention)
- Better and more accurate explanations of the processes of learning at a brain level than have been offered by some 'brain-friendly' teaching books in recent years
- Quick-to-read and easy-to-understand explanations that you can share with both children and colleagues

Neuron bits

It's your brain that allows you to laugh and cry, dance and sing, to solve life's daily problems and do all the other things you do. It can achieve this because of the amazing abilities of the billions of brain cells, or **neurons**, inside it. (If you were able to see your learners' brain cells and count them one by one, it would take you about 3000 years!)

These tiny little cells are the fundamental building blocks that allow their brains to work. Signals are passed between neurons by chemicals called **neurotransmitters**. Typically these travel from the **axon terminals** of one neuron to the **dendrites** of another across a tiny gap (or **synapse**) – although synapses can form in a wide range of ways. Neurotransmitters excite or inhibit the receiving brain cell. In turn, the next cell sends a spike of electricity down its **axon** and the process continues through the brain. **Myelin** insulates the axon and helps to regulate the flow of current. The result is a storm of electrical activity – and, as if by magic, you are you!

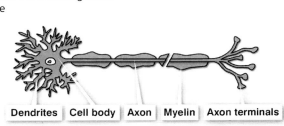

| Dendrites | Cell body | Axon | Myelin | Axon terminals |

Are your neurons excited by this?

Educators and brain scientists tend to have different working definitions of the word learning:

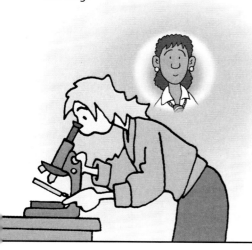

Some scientists working in laboratories judge learning by the excitability of groups of brain cells under a microscope; whereas educators judge learning in a slightly more traditional way – by the accumulation of knowledge and skills and/or levels of engagement. Neither is wrong: they are simply looking at things from different perspectives and using different methods.

Whichever way you look at it, learning requires the excitation of brain cells.

Getting those little grey cells excited

So how can you get your learners' brain cells excited so that learning happens more effectively? Ask yourself:

'What kinds of stimuli are most likely to excite the little grey cells and make them sit up and listen?'

In particular, remember that because human beings have evolved to be very sociable your learners' brains will more readily pay attention to information presented to them if linked to social processes.

For example, the important events in World War II will become more salient if presented from the perspective of the people involved or alive at the time, rather than if just stated as a list of facts, particularly if you create activities and discussions about such points of view. Get your students to imagine themselves and their families experiencing the war, for instance.

Connecting up

It is **interconnectivity** between neurons and across the brain that enables intelligence, effective memory function, physical abilities and skills. And, ultimately, it's interconnectivity that affects achievement. What to do about this:

- Ensure that you organise learning activities in your classroom in ways that provide opportunities for the connection of ideas
- Reward and praise children for making connections between different areas of learning and different topics
- Approach what you are teaching in a range of ways, with different types of sensory stimuli and a mixture of practical activity, thinking, conversation and reflection

This probably does not come as a surprise to you, but with this background knowledge perhaps you can feel more confident about challenging some of the more simplistic ideas about teaching and learning and feel justified in making your lessons even more active, fun and varied.

Picture this...

If you were able to look into a brain at the level of detail where you could observe the behaviour of **neurons** you would see that there are three stages to the forming of memories:

1. A **stimulus** (or event) triggers two neurons to fire together.

2. Further stimulation leads to a third neuron firing and a circuit is formed with the neurons linking with each other.

3. If the right level of stimulation continues, the three neurons become sensitive to each others' firing so that in the future if one fires all three will fire together.

4. The web of **interconnectivity** spreads through the brain as more connections are made.

This helps to explain why **repetition, association** and the interconnection of information are important aspects of effective learning and teaching.

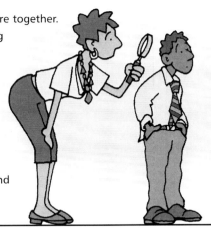

Differentiate

Interconnectivity in the brain is unique to each individual. Effective differentiation and the flexibility to adapt your teaching style and the materials you use to the needs of individual children may therefore be more than just philosophically sound ideas (from an educational equality point of view); they are probably essential for effective learning.

The ethical need to deliver effective differentiation is something that education research has long advocated from a qualitative and action research perspective and we can now begin to understand this from a scientific research perspective also. Furthermore, as we've already mentioned interconnectivity is also partly the result of your input and the way schools teach – which helps us to begin to see the interdependence and connections between things like social processes, brain science, learning theory and behaviour.

Grab them!

It stands to reason that if your learners' **neurons** start to switch off, your teaching won't be effective. To make neurons wake up and listen to you, the information that you deliver must be interpreted by the neurons to be **salient** and meaningful.

The brain has evolved so that it tunes into those things that may be important for its success and survival. In fact, you could say that it's constantly scanning the environment looking out for things that might like to eat it! Rather than bringing fearsome lions into the classroom to help you teach, try the following:

don't eat me!!

- The unexpected will always grab attention (at any age) and catching your learners off-guard in this way is guaranteed to make them remember an otherwise difficult lesson
- Things that are related to ourselves become instantly **salient**, so guide your learners towards using events in their own lives to help them remember things

Do it again and do it differently

It's not just a case of making information **salient** to make sure your pupils' neurons notice it. If you really want them to learn it, it's also important to **repeat** it.

But simple repetition is not enough. As we've seen, the brain likes **novelty** and **contrast** as well.

If you just repeat the same activities in the same way your pupils and their brains will become bored. Put another way, the brain will quickly notice that there is nothing new in the information and so pay less attention.

We'll talk more about **attention** later but for now let's see how repetition can stay exciting!

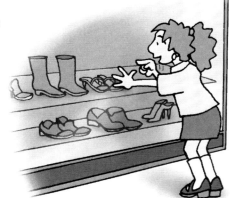

Impress that brain!

The brain can be literally unimpressed by repeated information that is no longer stimulating. To make sure this does not happen to your students' brains you can use rehearsal rather than repetition, coming up with novel ways of teaching the same information, eg:

- Teaching negative numbers by getting pupils to physically move up and down a line on the ground with zero in the middle
- Teaching foreign languages by inventing actions to go with the words, eg counting from 1-3 in Japanese can be accompanied by pupils acting out having an itchy knee and pointing to the sun:
  itchy = *'one' in Japanese*
  knee = *'two' in Japanese*
  sun = *'three' in Japanese*
- Making students teach the information to someone else or act out the sequence of events. (See next page.)

My students are neurons – sometimes

One way to teach your pupils what neurons are is to ask them to pretend to *be* neurons! Explain first about the parts of the neuron and which bits of their body will be those parts: the **dendrites** are like branches (fingers) and receive information, the **cell bodies** (head) process the information and the **axons** (legs) send it to the next neuron.

- Get all your pupils to lie head-to-toe on the floor with their legs together and hands by their ears (palms up, fingers outstretched, dendrite-like)'
- Every pupil should have some marbles by their feet
- Start the impulse off by rolling some marbles to the outstretched fingers of the first pupil
- When the marbles touch their fingers, their head should receive them with an accepting nod
- That pupil should then wiggle their body and legs before (gently!) using their feet to push their *own* marbles to the next person's fingers

Well, if it's good enough for biological psychology undergraduates it's good enough for Y9! It works at all levels!

The more you do it, the more you get

The more you learn, the better you get at learning. Because learning involves the creation of new connections between networks of neurons across the brain, the more you learn the fitter your brain becomes – just as with exercise generally. Things you can do with your students:

- Encourage them to seek out learning opportunities within and outside the classroom and to recognise opportunities for learning in the school external environment (eg collecting real leaves for a biology lesson rather than just drawing leaf pictures)
- Set more open-ended problems where students are really challenged to think and apply their existing knowledge; and ask more open questions
- Challenge their mental dexterity with a few quick-fire quizzes and increasingly demanding memory tasks – but remember to keep it fun

Just think about it

The power of thought is often underestimated: just thinking about something changes the structure of your brain. This was put to the test in a famous scientific study:

People were given one of three different tasks to investigate how the brain's wiring might change by learning to play the piano:

- One group just stared at a piano for several hours each day for five days
- The second group did simple five-finger piano exercises
- The third was asked to *imagine* performing the exercises

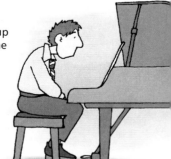

After the five days, the subjects' brains were scanned. The group who stared at the piano showed no changes. However, both the 'playing' and 'imagining' group showed identically large increases in the proportion of their brain used for their fingers.

Many athletes now visualise their performances to help 'train their brain' and teachers say that visualisation can help with learning in the classroom. Now you know why.

Neurons are always on the go

So, just thinking can change your brain. In fact, **neurons** are constantly moving in the early development of the brain. In the womb new neurons are grown all the time and some travel from the inner structures of the brain to outer layers along long fibres – a bit like riding a monorail. **Migration** takes between two and three weeks.

Neurons navigate using chemical signals released by outer brain layers. These help them to find their way – if the signals stop so does the migration.

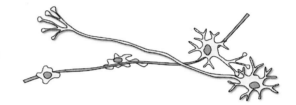

Although this sort of radical migration doesn't take place in later brain development, nonetheless neurons are constantly moving about, snuggling up to each other to make denser networks where they are needed or moving their dendrites and terminals (the little arm-like bits) about. This movement we now know takes place in response to the external environment and, of course, that includes the learning experiences that you create in the classroom.

How motivation works

Motivation also underpins effective learning and memory. We saw earlier that all your basic desires arise from your midbrain and limbic system and when followed through produce lovely, rewarding, positive emotions.

- Rewards help shape behaviour as you're more likely to choose to do things that you enjoy, so-called 'reward-seeking'
- Your **midbrain** gives you these pleasurable emotions, specifically through the release of a chemical called **dopamine**
- Though you might not think it, almost everything you choose to do comes with a reward and the release of dopamine. When you finally decide to eat that chocolate cake, the reward is immediate! But when you choose to take out a pension plan, the reward is a long way off

So 'catch the children doing the right thing' by noticing what they are doing that you like, mentioning it, and in doing so rewarding their behaviour. The more you do this the more you increase the likelihood of them doing the right thing again. As the education research describes it, have a **continuous schedule of positive reward**.

Mood in the classroom

A change in the levels of a brain chemical called **serotonin**, which is important in mood, affects learning. Higher levels of serotonin, as with positive mood, make people less sensitive to negative feedback and more sensitive to positive feedback; lower serotonin, as with negative mood, leads to the opposite effect. We now know that:

* Those in a positive mood rely on existing knowledge and are over-confident in their abilities
* Those in a negative mood rely only on what they are presented with for the task, may be more systematic and analytical, and lack confidence in their abilities

Therefore, you might find that certain tasks are done better in certain moods. For instance, more creative activities may be better performed in a positive mood whilst solving difficult mathematical problems might be better done in a less excited frame of mind.

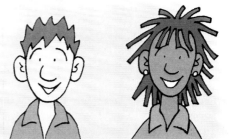

Stay awake but don't get stressed!

There is a complex relationship between the levels of **arousal** of your pupils, or how ready they are to engage with something, and how efficiently they will learn. You can see from the graph that at low levels of arousal (barely awake and not paying attention) they will learn very little. However, at the high levels of arousal associated with stress they will also learn very little.

- Arousal is associated with **noradrenalin** release in the brain which can help your neurons make the connections needed to learn and form memories

- At high levels of sustained arousal, seen with stress, hormones are released that can cause the dendrites of your **hippocampal** neurons to wither, making it impossible to form the new connections you need to learn

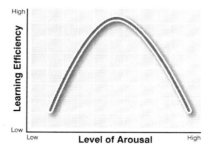

As a teacher, you need to carefully modulate your pupils' levels of arousal by keeping them engaged and attentive whilst also preventing stress levels running high.

The Neuroscience of Memory

What is memory?

From a neuroscience point of view, learning is the process whereby neurons that fire together in response to an experience are altered in a way that means that they will fire together again in the future:

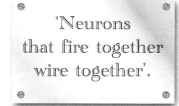

'Neurons that fire together wire together'.

The repeated and combined firing of neurons is what makes you **remember** something. In fact, the very process of recalling something makes the neurons that fired together more likely to do the same thing in the future.

Continually repeating an experience makes it easier to remember – if you do it in interesting and stimulating ways! This is why in the classroom you must remember to:

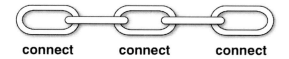

connect   connect   connect

Are you paying attention?

So is that it then – just repeating stuff – is that all you have to do to learn things well? Well no, because **attention** has a big effect on learning and retention too. As we said earlier, the brain is constantly scanning the environment for dangers to our survival. It is the process of attention that controls and directs what we are aware of – like a sort of highlighting pen that makes things stand out.

Attentional processes select the things that the brain thinks are most important and amplify how we respond to that stimulus. In the classroom you can attract attention:

- With a single input (visual, auditory, bodily sensations) if it is striking enough
- With more than one modality input (ie a fun activity involving all senses)
- By building curiosity at the start of a lesson – particularly important because of the **primacy effect**, ie remembering the first thing in a learning episode (see page 86)

Go on… … let your creativity run wild!

Different types of attention

Although **attention** is often thought of as one thing, there are actually a number of different types of attention:

1. **Selective** –The ability to maintain attention to a particular thing even in the presence of distractions.
2. **Alternating** –The ability to shift attention focus between tasks.
3. **Focused** –The ability to respond to specific stimuli only.
4. **Sustained** –The ability to maintain attention during continuous and repetitive activity.
5. **Divided** –The highest level of attention, referring to the ability to respond simultaneously to multiple tasks or multiple task demands.

In the classroom make sure that you are providing opportunities for your students to use all types of attention so that you support them to develop their full range of learning skills. It's easy to slip into one approach if you are not careful.

Implications for the classroom

The processes of **attention** are a good example of where the neuroscience evidence can help us to understand why certain things that we know to be good practice are so important in the classroom. Things like:

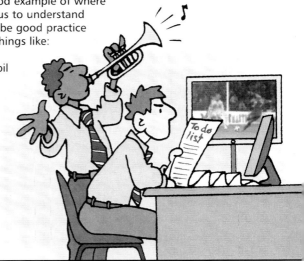

- Setting clear tasks where the pupil knows exactly what to do
- Keeping distractions to a minimum
- Giving indications of how long learners will need to work on the task
- Giving breaks if necessary

Attention and learning

To sum up so far, we've seen that:

1. For information to be learnt, your neurons must think that it is **salient** (novel, relevant, noticeable and attention-grabbing) and they must experience it repeatedly.
2. This **repetition**, however, must be offset against boredom because the brain must pay attention to a stimulus if it is going to learn about it.
3. One way to help pupils pay attention to the stimulus is to **rehearse** it in different ways rather than repeat it in the same way.

On the next page you will see an example that illustrates just how powerful attention can be as a mediator of learning.

Inattention blindness

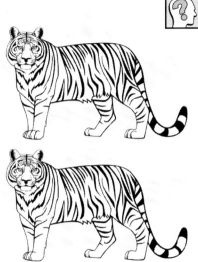

When our attention is focused on an image, or something that we are looking at, it's easy to be deceived into thinking that we're seeing all of the information that is there.

Look at the two images on the right. Most people will have to scan both pictures in a methodical way to spot the differences. They won't be able to notice them with just a glance. This is called **inattention blindness**. Usually, we pay enough attention only to the big or unusual parts of an image.

Psychologist Dan Simons provides some good demonstrations of inattention blindness at: http://viscog.beckman.illinois.edu/djs_lab/demos.html.

Paying better attention

In the classroom you can counteract **inattention blindness** by:

- Being careful about the amount of information you give in one go. Just because you know all the details doesn't mean that your students' attentional processes can deal with it all in one go the first time they see it
- Teach children about inattention blindness with some fun activities (like the one on the previous page) that help them learn to be methodical with large scale new information
- Be particularly careful to avoid jumping around in explanations of content
- Break topics down into small memorable chunks
- Avoid giving too many instructions at once

The next step on from attention is the process of **working memory**. Working memory is quite limited and so you need to give it the best possible chance to be effective.

Working and long-term memory

As you may already know, memory can be broken down into short-term and long-term stores both of which involve encoding, storing and retrieving information. The term **working memory** has now replaced the old ideas of short-term memory and although it is still shorter lasting than long-term memory, it is quite flexible as you will see later on.

	Working memory	Episodic buffer	Long-term memory
How is it stored?	Active rehearsal	*Holding space linking working and long-term memory*	Passive storage
How long does it last?	A few seconds		Days, years, lifetime
How big is the store?	About seven items		Infinite

Stages in forming a working memory

Although all experiences affect our brains, some can enter our **working memory** (which is only a temporary holding place) through a series of steps:

- **Attention** is drawn to something very quickly, causing activity in all the sensory areas of the brain
- An emotional response may also occur, involving brain areas such as the **amygdala**
- If the stimulus is sufficiently **salient** it will enter our working memory, which is known to involve part of the **forebrain** called the **prefrontal cortex**
- It will only remain in working memory while you work to keep it there – a bit like writing in the sand – after each wave you will need to go over it or it will disappear

Find out what some of the implications of this are for learning and teaching on the next page.

How limited is working memory?

Research in the 1950s by one of the founders of cognitive psychology, George Miller, suggested that **working memory** may only be able to process seven (plus or minus two) pieces of information at once.

More recent research, supported by neuroscience evidence, suggests that it may in fact usually be far less than that. Some people suggest that one piece of information is probably as much as is possible in certain situations. What to do about this:

- Make sure you engage your learners and get their attention
- Be careful how many instructions you give at once. Keep it to no more than three steps or stages if the learning process is a new one
- Emotions and personal relevance can enhance entrance to working memory. So make sure the information is relevant and connects with your learners before you as< questions

Chunking

You can maximise your working memory capacity by **chunking** information together into meaningful categories for rehearsal, eg:

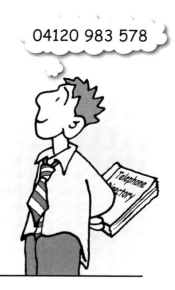

04120 983 578

- Chunk information according to category, eg food items in a shopping list, or members of the same family

- Make a string of numbers meaningful by joining them together in a certain way, for example: 0 1 8 7 5 2 4 8 6 5 9 could be chunked to the dialling code 01875 and two chunks of three 248 and 659

By creating meaningful chunks of information you can combine lots of smaller items and keep them in your working memory more easily.

More ways to chunk information

On the previous page we saw how we could chunk information by breaking large amounts of information into smaller bite-sized pieces. This type of chunking is sometimes called **pattern chunking**. You can use pattern chunking by making up a story about a series of otherwise unrelated objects that you want to remember, eg DOG, RIVER, BALL, BOY, BAT, BEE:

The DOG *jumped into the* RIVER *to fetch a* BALL *that the* BOY *hit there with his* BAT *because a* BEE *distracted him*

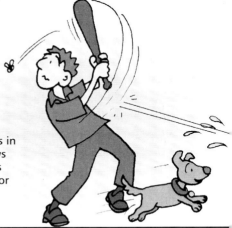

The more sophisticated form of chunking is **categorical chunking** where you get learners to group information into simpler categories (perhaps in a table or a mind map). For example: *advantages* vs *disadvantages*; *structure* vs *function*; *differences* vs *similarities*. When you list things by size or shape, or use taxonomies, you are doing something similar.

The 'hands up trap'

Because **working memory** is only a temporary holding space you can easily be tricked into thinking that students have learnt something if you just ask a couple of quick questions after presenting some new information (what you might call the 'hands up trap').

Just because the information was held in working memory doesn't mean it got any further in the learning process. Also, just because something is in one child's working memory doesn't mean it is in anyone else's. So avoid the 'hands up trap' in the following ways:

- Use more challenging higher order questions that require the *use* of the facts you have presented and not just the *repetition* of those facts
- Target individual children with questions rather than allowing just anyone to answer

From working to long-term memory

It is not quite clear *how* working memory is stored in the **prefrontal cortex**, but long-term memory information is thought to be stored through **plasticity**, ie the changes in the connections within the brain. Entrance to long-term memory also occurs in stages:

- Meaningful stimuli from working memory move into long-term memory, involving a structure called the **hippocampus**

- Other brain regions may become more active as the memory is consolidated with memory stored across brain regions – rather like a network of filing cabinets

Take a moment to re-read this chapter and think about the importance of high levels of **stimulation**, **attention**, **association** and **repetition** in your classroom practice.

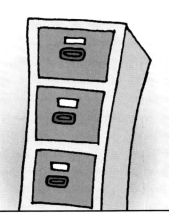

Types of long-term memory

As we have seen memory can be divided into **working memory** and **long-term memory**. Long-term memory can be broken down into a number of forms beginning with **declarative memory** and **procedural memory**.

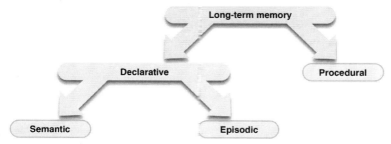

1. **Declarative memory** refers to knowledge that you can declare and this in itself breaks down into **semantic** and **episodic** memories.

2. **Semantic** knowledge refers to facts about the world whilst **episodic** refers to autobiographical knowledge (episodes of personal experience).

3. **Procedural memory** refers to things we can *do* rather than *declare*, eg riding a bike.

Semantic memory

Teachers deal with semantic memory everyday. This is memory about meaning and of recollection of factual information and knowledge about the world.

Your memory contains information for particular categories and has individual items linked to these categories. For example, a robin will match up with many of the properties associated with the category of bird and therefore you recognise it as a bird.

You can think of your memory as a network of information – a bit like a train or tube map – and the bigger the network the stronger the memory. Since the size of the network is important, you should always try to build new information onto older, established networks so that it can access the strength of existing, related memories. Also, you should make the categories for organising the information explicit (which is why mind mapping can be helpful).

Episodic memory

Episodic memory is autobiographical. Like semantic memory, it can still be considered a network, but it is easier to remember information about yourself than it is to remember information about an historical fact or figure. This is because:

- You have a very large network of information about yourself in your brain – you are an expert on you!
- Events in your own life tend to be accompanied by strong emotions, such as your birthday or wedding day
- Events can also be accompanied by negative emotions and these memories are equally persistent

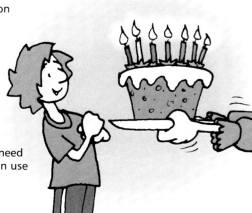

As a teacher, although you will not necessarily need to access your pupils' **episodic** memory, you can use it to help their **semantic** memory.

Using episodic memory to enhance semantic memory

1. We know that information about ourselves is always more meaningful than anything else and that to help improve our memory we should make things more meaningful.
2. Because the network in our brains for 'us' is so strong, if we link to this network we can strengthen our memory for other things. This is called **self-referencing**.

To self-reference, ask someone to relate what they need to learn to themselves. For instance, ask them to look at a list of colours and think about which ones they like. They will remember the list better than if you just asked them to read it – even if they did not like the colours!

You can see these two ideas in action on the next few pages.

It means so much more

To illustrate the effect of giving meaning to the things you want to learn, let's do a quick memory test. Below is a list of words. Read the list, looking to see whether each word contains the letter 'e'. Cover the list up, wait one minute and then try to write down all the items of the list.

car	lion	pickle	tank	pencil
lemon	motorway	banana	elephant	class
home	bottle	apron	egg	basket
potato	knife	brush	computer	cloud

Now, read the list below, this time thinking which items you might find in a kitchen. As before, cover the list up, wait one minute and write down as many as you can remember. Make a note of how well you did on each list.

tree	cat	kettle	monkey	cloth
apple	bowl	laptop	cereal	moon
caravan	table	oven	toaster	hairbrush
fork	bed	petrol	stapler	condiments

It's all about me

On the previous tests it is likely that you found you remembered more of the second list because you had to *process the meaning* of the words (ie you had to think more about them).

Now let's test the self-referencing idea. Read the list of human characteristics below, thinking about whether they are positive or negative traits. Cover it up, wait one minute and try to write as many down as you can remember.

kind	generous	grumpy	conniving	tidy
jolly	moody	funny	hard-working	outgoing
two-faced	gentle	loyal	lazy	shy

Now read through the next list of adjectives thinking about whether or not they apply to you.

sad	extrovert	conscientious	noisy	open
timid	amusing	sweet	firm	honest
happy	manipulative	sharing	fair	messy

You probably remembered more of the second list because you linked it to you!

Implications

So what are the implications of neuroscience for learning and teaching? In our view, the neuroscience evidence does not contradict the teacher effectiveness research. Rather, it helps to provide a further explanation of the key attributes of highly effective teachers* and what they do, particularly in relation to areas such as:

- Ensuring **challenge**
- Maintaining high levels of **engagement**
- Having high levels of **social interaction**
- Using **questioning** effectively
- Communicating high teacher **expectations**
- Creating a **positive emotional atmosphere**
- **Subject knowledge** – your learners' brains can only work in response to the quality of the information they are given!

Take a moment to think about your own practice as a teacher and which of the areas above you most need to develop. Then go on to read the next section. This will give you more tips and ideas about how to develop your practice further.

*For more about teacher effectiveness research read *Effective Teaching: evidence and practice* by Dr Daniel Muijs and Prof David Reynolds. Sage Publications Ltd, 2001

Introduction

 Brain Bits

 The Learning Process

 The Neuroscience of Memory

 In the Classroom ◀

 The Developing Brain

 Future Issues for Brain Science in the Classroom

 Reflective Summary

In the Classroom

What's in this section?

This section contains a wide range of tips and strategies to enhance learning and memory in the classroom. We begin by looking at what can go wrong with memory and what you can do about it. This is followed by a brief discussion of some common 'neuro-myths' and what neuroscience really says about these ideas.

We return again to working memory, this time looking at its structure and what that can tell us about learning. There are several pages dealing with lesson structure and how this can be improved to enhance learning.

Finally, we cover some more general information on, for instance, creativity and consciousness and finish by looking at a range of particular needs such as dyslexia, ADHD and teaching gifted and talented students.

Things that can go wrong with memory

1. Focusing on the wrong things

Sometimes the process of memory can be undermined. The next few pages describe some of the ways this can happen and what you can do about it.

The brain constantly works to store things that might be useful later, letting other things pass it by. However, if **attention** is not focused on the right things, information may be coded badly in the first place (like remembering the colour of someone's hair but not their actual face). What to do:

- Make explicit to learners the thing that is most important
- Excite neurons by making this area interesting, and use repetition for reinforcement but beware of boring the brain into a lack of attention again

Things that can go wrong with memory

2. Confusing similar concepts

We have all experienced learners jumbling up similar but different concepts when they come to doing a test. Although making associations is a really good idea in the classroom, think carefully about the associations you're going to build into the learning so that you don't lead your learners' brains to connect things in the wrong way.

Those things that are selected for memory are stored in association with pre-existing memories. This means that items can sometimes get misfiled. What to do:

• Organise the way you teach logically, with meaningful categories that are easy to recall

• Create connections and interconnectivity – with other curriculum areas and within aspects of a subject – in ways that help learners to solve problems and think carefully about the information they are using

Things that can go wrong with memory

3. Forgetting and false memories

The brain forgets information almost as soon as it has remembered it. This is why it's important in lessons to return regularly to previous learning, even when the topic is unrelated. So, rather than leaving revision until the end of the year, make it a constant part of your lesson planning.

In addition, every time we remember something there is the potential for the memory to change. Sometimes this can improve the quality of the memory but other times alterations can create **false memories**.

When revising, do so thoroughly. Don't be tempted just to skip over the surface; make sure that you have given the topic sufficient depth in relation to understanding key processes, concepts and facts, even if you have reduced the content covered.

Things that can go wrong with memory

4. Tip of the tongue

Tip of the tongue, another natural phenomenon, is familiar to all of us: that inability to recall something despite great certainty that it is known. So far there is no one clear explanation of this from a brain science perspective. However, here are some suggestions about what to do when it happens to learners in the classroom:

- Stop and come back to it later after doing something completely different
- Give the learner the chance to be rewarded again later when they can remember it
- Avoid implying fault or punishment when this happens – you risk conditioning 'fight' or 'flight' reactions in your students when you are questioning them, whereas you need their prefrontal cortex, and therefore working memory, to be 'up for the job'

Beware of 'neuro-myths'

You may be surprised not to be reading lots about VAK, learning styles, brain gym and differences in how boys and girls learn in this book. They don't appear because there is no neuroscience evidence to support many of the 'brain-based' explanations that have been created to justify activities associated with these types of areas. (See following page.)

However, that doesn't mean you should discount such activities. Brain science isn't saying don't do something if you, as a teacher, know it works – just to remember that not everything needs an invented neuroscience explanation. Take PowerPoint – there is no neuroscience evidence for its effectiveness and you don't need to invent some brain science explanation to justify it. You just know that sometimes it helps you teach.

The science bit

So what *does* neuroscience tell us about some of the areas mentioned on the previous page?

- **VAK** – varied sensory input is good. However, it is important to realise that the whole brain is active all the time and sensory brain areas do not operate in isolation. Although people may feel that they have preferences, as far as the brain is concerned all sensory areas work together. What you are probably experiencing when you are consciously aware of the effect of visual and auditory stimuli are the different parts of working memory (the visual cache and phonological store). We will discuss these in a minute

- **Brain gym** – a small amount of exercise can improve short-term memory and a fun activity can be very motivating. However, brain gym doesn't integrate the 'left and right halves' of the brain. This happens all the time without any outside help!

- **'Left and right brained'** – there is no research evidence to support the idea that someone is left or right brained. The whole brain is active all the time in everyone

- **Girls' brains and boys' brains** are not significantly different at the level of brain science that is important in memory and retention

The structure of working memory

The structure of working memory is relevant to the classroom because you trigger different components depending on what sort of input and tasks you give learners.

Central executive – neither visual nor auditory and allocates resources to the other parts of working memory.

Visual cache (or visuo-spatial sketch pad) – like a temporary whiteboard holding visual and spatial information. It includes an inner scribe that can picture writing and drawing.

Phonological store (or loop) – allows rehearsal of acoustic information and includes a process for hearing words in your head (your inner speech). The loop deals with verbal material and can preserve the order of information as it goes round and round.

Episodic buffer – integrates information and can store both visual and acoustic information.

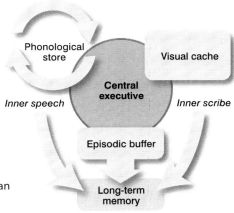

Some of working memory's components

On the previous page we talked about the components of working memory. You can experience the usefulness of these different functions by doing the following:

1. First, just by saying the names of the days of the week in order in your head, try to work out what would be the 11th day after Wednesday. (Don't use visual inner imaginings or other strategies to help you get there.)

Some people will experience how nearly impossible it is for your phonological store (inner voice) to say the days of the week and count at the same time.

2. Now this time, as you say the days of the week to yourself, imagine hanging the names onto pegs labelled 1-11.

You will probably find it quite easy to visualise at the same time. This may be the reason why it is more effective for many people to learn languages by doing more than just hearing them (for instance, visualising and writing as well).

Get even more from working memory

We've seen that working memory contains an '**episodic buffer**' (a sort of holding space) which links to **long-term** memory. Getting information to this stage and out of the temporary store of **working memory** is essential for retention. Try these ideas:

- Trigger the buffer by finding ways of presenting the information that directly relate to children's experience and by giving novel and imaginative 'episodes' of experiential learning related to the information (eg take them outside the classroom to look at the angles and shapes of the school building as part of a maths lesson, giving them the opportunity to identify and measure their own examples of acute and obtuse angles)
- Present information in a variety of ways to ensure repetition
- Ask questions that relate the information to previous learning by probing for understanding and thinking
- Use discussion and group work and get your students to teach each other about what they found
- Don't present information just visually or just verbally; find ways to do both at the same time

Lesson structure and memory 1

The Von Restorff effect

So how can you plan lessons that will improve your chances of getting stuff from fickle old **working memory** into **long-term** memory?

When it comes to sensory input, brain science shows that all primates are predominantly visual.

You can tap into this potential resource by using plenty of visual content to help to stimulate attention, learning and memory. So make more use of:

- Visual imagery and metaphor
- Storytelling and visualisations
- Colourful mind mapping with visual images to sum up ideas

That the single most memorable and unusual image in a mass of other data is likely to be the most remembered thing was first noted in the 1930s by the psychologist **Hedwig von Restorff** – no, not the owl in Harry Potter.

Lesson structure and memory 2

Cuddly toy, fondue set, kettle, cuddly toy

Whenever you're given a long list of things to remember, no doubt – like everyone else – you'll not be able to remember every item. The chances are, though, that the item you're most likely to recall will be very predictable.

To demonstrate this, try to remember the objects in the single list alongside by spending a second or two on each before moving on to the next word. Only read the list once! Then stop, close the book and write down what you remember. Then turn to the next page.

Apple
Wristwatch
Umbrella
Plantpot
Plate
Potato
Teddybear
Keys
Spoon
Screwdriver
Peach
Knife
Saucer
Wallet
Phone
Carrot
Toy

Lesson structure and memory 3

First and last things

You're much more likely to remember the first and last items but forget ones in the middle – because your brain is paying more attention at the start and the later items are not crowded in your memories with any subsequent ones. Did you find this?

The graph shows the proportion of words that a group recalled when given a similar list to those on the previous page.

This is known as the **primacy** and **recency** effect. It means extra effort must be applied during *the middle* of lessons (or any learning episode) to boost attention if learning is to take place.

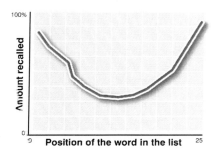

Lesson structure and memory 4

Implications for the classroom

How to use the information from the last few pages in the classroom:

1. Structure lessons with a number of shorter **episodes** so there are more high points of retention. Although there will be dips, you will avoid that long low period in the middle.

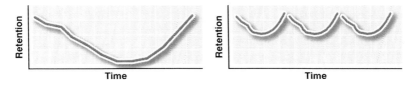

2. Apply some of the other principles discussed earlier by making sure that your first and last piece of input is presented in an interesting and novel way and that these moments contain summaries of the most important information.

Lesson structure and memory 5

Association and connection

As we know, **interconnectivity** is also essential for effective learning, so add **associations**, **repetition** and interconnectivity to each learning episode and between episodes (especially in the middle).

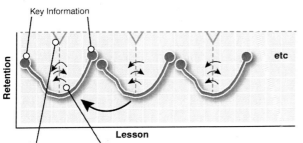

Key Information

Retention

Lesson

Striking and unusual image that sums up the learning episode

Associations, connections and repetition

You could also add a **Von Restorff** image to each episode, ie a single striking unusual image that sums up the learning for that episode (see page 84). Do more association and repetition, and have your Von Restorff in the middle of the learning episode when retention is likely to be at it lowest!

Of course, this is not a magic formula; you will need to use your professional skills to apply the principles differently for different topics – but you get the idea.

Lesson structure and memory 6

Motivation

Motivation is also key to retention and memory so ensure that your learners can relate what you are teaching to where they are coming from and to their interests. You can increase the **salience** (attention-grabbing nature) of the content you teach by making it personally meaningful and relevant to your students and you can improve general motivation by maintaining a positive emotional climate and by using frequent specific praise to reinforce the behaviours that you want to see again. **Humour** is also a great motivator.

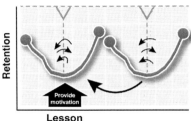

Now take a few minutes to look back over the last few pages on lesson structure and memory. Notice how we have practised what we preach and in our explanation made use of the same principles described here. Look for the different elements, starting on page 84 and the Von Restorff effect. (Answers overleaf.)

Lesson structure and memory 7

Here's what we did:
- We introduced **Von Restorff** first and came to **motivation** last as these are really key pieces of information (**primacy and recency effect**). You will have noticed the Harry Potter image also!
- The whole learning is summed up with a single striking visual (diagram on page 88)
- **Association** and **repetition** were used as we built up the diagram
- Everything was referred back to the classroom and your practice, making a connection to where you are coming from (**salience**)
- By getting you to read this answer we summed it all up again and made a final use of the **recency** effect.
- Having to look back over the pages added another sensory input as will the next task

Next:
See how easy it is to draw the diagram yourself and label it without looking!
Then go and tell someone else about it.
How could you do something similar in your next lesson?

Categories and learning

The moment that we put a piece of information into a category our brains will begin to stop paying as much attention to the stimulus. For example, when you see a cat and you label it 'cat' in your brain you will no longer take in all the detail.

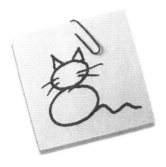

This is one of the reasons we can often be surprised in the classroom when we think we have covered something and in fact we haven't done it as well as we thought. (Of course, sometimes the kids just weren't listening!)

Frequent use of good higher order questions may well be important for teacher effectiveness because it forces your students' brains to return to a stimulus, exploring it from more varied perspectives until the full detail begins to move from working memory to long-term memory.

You can think too much...

On the last page we saw how categorising can lead to editing out details. The **pre-frontal cortex** manages this sort of editing or generalising process. There is some evidence to suggest that turning *off* some thinking processes gives a greater potential to be creative. (Have you ever found yourself thinking so hard you make mistakes?) Therefore, just as it is important to focus attention in the classroom, it is equally important to provide opportunities for spontaneous, non-thinking activities. For example:

• Asking really 'big picture' open questions about a topic

• Getting students to create a metaphor or symbol that relates to their learning

• When engaged in learning activities that contain detailed knowledge, ensure breaks (eg get your students to talk to each other between sets of descriptions or to engage in a fun revision activity such as walking round the room and when the music stops getting them to ask the person next to them the revision question on a card they've been given, swap cards and carry on)

Remember **working memory** is a sort of sketch and has very limited capacity, so filling it with more detail when a child is stuck on a concept may simply compound the issue.

Being on autopilot

We often talk about being on autopilot. A lot of what happens in the brain happens automatically, without conscious awareness. This is true not only for simple tasks but for well-learned complex ones.

Imagine a footballer about to head a cross. The process begins in the brain with attention. Within milli-seconds this triggers further unconscious steps (eg action planning and the sending of signals). Conscious thought doesn't start until right at the end of the process and it is only at this point that the football player in our example has the conscious awareness of action needed. With practice our player develops better and better unconscious actions and there will be less need to override these.

Early in the learning process this triggering of conscious thought too late can be very frustrating, particularly for children with problems such as ADHD.

Ladders

One great way to explain the implications of unconscious action and learning to learners is by using a model that is often talked about in education: the 4-rung ladder of learning.

Some people even add a fifth stage: 'conscious mastery' – the ability to carry out perfect tasks automatically with high levels of consciousness – where you can demonstrate and teach to others.

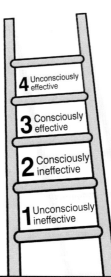

- Explain the model to your students and get them to relate it to a real life example of something they now do automatically without having to think about it
- Get them to fold their arms and then do it the other way (the uncomfortable way). Repeat lots of times and ask them what they notice (the more repetitions the easier it gets – and quite quickly)
- Point out where they are on the ladder in relation to a task or the learning of facts, concepts and processes and praise their persistence in moving forward – you can always replace the word 'effective' with the more child-friendly 'successful'

Doing two things at once

Asking learners to do a new, complex thinking task while still doing another can lead brain functioning to stall. This may be because the **prefrontal cortex**, responsible for redirecting attention from one situation to another, can't do this instantly. However, brains can do similar things at once (eg, listening to someone talking whilst reading).

Try to rotate one arm clockwise whilst rotating a foot anticlockwise (dancers can do this but most people can't). Compare it to rotating both in the same direction.

- As a teacher, ask yourself if the two things that need to be done really need to be done at once
- When you set up a task make sure students end it cleanly and are ready to move on
- In learning processes with several steps, be clear with your instructions and explain if you want pupils to focus on a single type of learning process first (ending this before moving on) so they don't try to engage in both similar complex tasks at once

Attention vs conscious thought

You will have noticed the way in which we use the words 'attention' and 'conscious thought' differently in this book. It is quite an important distinction from a brain science point of view and one that teachers are sometimes unaware of.

Attention is a process that happens in response to a stimulus and can be at the level of unconscious action. It happens very early in the processes of memory and behaviour.

Conscious thought happens very late in the process (some would argue far too late to be the controlling mechanism) and, unless things have been learnt to a high level, has limited ability to influence the behaviour that is just at that moment happening.

Begin to recognise that much of what you have communicated has had an effect at an automatic unconscious level before your pupils have conscious awareness of it. Be sure you have attracted their attention – have clear routines and simple signals for getting the class to stop work quickly – as well as having their conscious awareness!

Practice makes perfect

If you're the kind of educator who is always telling your learners that time spent practising a skill is time well spent, and that determination and patience pay off, then prepare for some robust neuroscience evidence that will back you up!

Have you ever tried to juggle? If so, you'll know how difficult it is to co-ordinate your arms and eyes and body position to make three small balls move smoothly through the air exactly where you want them to go. If you've never tried, it's easy to imagine how tricky it is!

However, if you practise juggling every day, your brain will actually start to grow as your performance improves! This has been shown to be the case in young adults as well as in people aged around 75 years. As you might expect, the growth will be mainly in the bits of your brain that control your limbs and co-ordinate your body. By learning a new skill you can grow your brain!

In fact, just thinking about doing something (see page 46) can have remarkable effects on your brain.

Modelling and mimicking

The size of your **cortex** makes you very different from other creatures. It also contains specialised neurons that are tuned-in to social interaction. The cortex helps you use reason and logic to solve problems and plan ahead. It may have developed in response to living in complex social groups.

Some neurons in your cortex **(mirror neurons)** activate not just when you make particular movements but also when you see someone else making movements, leading to an unconscious mimicking of other people's actions.

Many people believe that this process is fundamental to the process of learning. It may help to explain the power of modelling tasks and activities in the classroom – as you demonstrate, the brains of your children are instantly, and unconsciously, mimicking your actions ready to perform the task themselves.

So look for opportunities to model how to learn and identify the key activities that experts in your subject do. Point out these processes when you do them and get the children to observe each other as they in turn model, noticing and feeding back on improvements.

Attention Deficit Hyperactivity Disorder

ADHD is a very common disorder in children and is characterised by poor attention, hyperactivity and impulsiveness. It is now known to persist into adulthood in about 60% of individuals. Despite having reasonably effective treatment, normally medication, we do not fully understand what causes ADHD and what changes in the brain might occur. However, here is some of what we do know:

- Compared to children without ADHD, those with the disorder have an overall reduction in brain size as well as reduced volumes of some specific regions
- There is lots of evidence from individuals with ADHD compared to healthy individuals to suggest that changes occur in the function of a brain chemical called **dopamine**
- Dopamine is involved in responding to reward

Effective drug treatments increase levels of dopamine and **noradrenalin**.

ADHD – what to do in the classroom

Children with ADHD may show particular problems in:

- Working memory and planning but these can occur in children without ADHD as well
- Resisting an immediate small reward to gain a larger reward later on

There are a number of things you can do to help children with ADHD in your classroom:

- Reduce reliance on working memory and help them make plans
- Where working memory is essential, use some of the strategies you read earlier to help them maximise their memory

To encourage them to delay 'cashing in' and instead work towards a long-term goal, give them plenty of filler activities to do whilst they wait.

(See *Challenging Behaviours Pocketbook* for more information on ADHD.)

Dyslexia

Dyslexia is the commonest learning disability. People with dyslexia have difficulty in learning to read, regardless of all other talents and despite average or above average intelligence. Reading difficulty is often associated with problems linking particular phonemes with their correct letters.

- Dyslexia can run in families
- It is thought that the genes that tell neurons where they should be when they migrate in the brain don't work properly
- The brain areas important in processing and producing language are underactive in many dyslexics during reading
- There are alterations in the connections between these brain areas

Dyslexia can often be effectively treated through school-based reading interventions that can even reverse the underactivity in language areas that were initially observed. Some neuroscientists think that eating fish oils may help with axon flexibility, other people suggest coloured glasses – but as yet there is no clear winner in relation to the best strategy, so keep doing what you find works.

(See the *Dyslexia Pocketbook* for more information.)

Autism

Children with autism have difficulties in communicating and with social relationships. They show inflexibility and repetitiveness in interests and actions. The extent to which these difficulties occur varies considerably, which is why it is more appropriate to refer to the 'autism spectrum' than simply 'autism'.

Neuroscience research is only one of many types of research into this spectrum but it has revealed some interesting findings:

- The **synapse** (gap between two neurons) does not function normally
- Regulation of the brain chemical **serotonin** is altered in some autistic people
- Low levels of the hormone **oxytocin** are found in people with autism – this is thought to be especially important in social relationships

Currently there is no one accepted theory but a number of areas are being explored.

Autism – what to do in the classroom

The changes in the brain identified above have not led to any direct interventions for the classroom. However, we do know that children on the autistic spectrum may have problems planning and can be hypersensitive to sensory stimuli. You can help them in these areas by providing a clear structure, eg:

- Use a daily planner of activities
- Use visual reminders to keep them on task
- Avoid distractions from previous activities such as older instructions written on the white board

Structure can also be provided in the physical and sensory environment:

- Have well-defined spaces for specific tasks (with visual symbols indicating task)
- Reduce busy visual patterns and background noise

The highly able brain

Some education writers (eg John Geake*) have drawn on neuroscience evidence to point to the idea that very talented learners have developed more interconnectivity in their brains. This in turn enables better executive functioning (what the front wrinkly bit – the **prefrontal cortex** – does), focused attention and working memory. Here are some suggestions for ways to support such learners and keep them motivated:

Include more activities involving high memory demands

Give feedback so learners know what they are good at and to stop them underestimating their higher level skills

Include more analysis and synthesis in topics

Give fewer small repetitive tasks

Extend the curriculum and make connections explicit

**The Brain at School: Educational Neuroscience in the Classroom* by John Geake, Open University Press, 2009.

The Developing Brain

Bursting brains

When you were born you were entirely reliant on your family to feed you and keep you warm and safe. This is because your brain took a great deal of time to fully develop – longer than the brain of any other animal on the planet. In fact, it would not have been fully mature by the time you left school.

It isn't that you have grown more brain cells – you were born with almost all the brain cells you have now. Growth has been the result of massive increases in the numbers of connections between those cells. At its peak, your brain was creating over 40,000 connections per second and, as a result, is now four times the size it was when you were born!

A lot of this growth happens thanks to a basic brain blueprint but childhood environment also has a part to play. The cortex is wrinkly because as it has evolved there has literally not been enough space for its vast surface area.

What's in this section:

① The major milestones in brain development:
- Childhood
- Adolescence
- Adulthood

② How teaching practices can match the development of learners' brains

Hot heads – the young child's brain

What is your earliest memory? Chances are it will be from when you were 3-4 years old because the part of the brain important for long-term memories (the **hippocampus**) becomes highly developed at this time. Your memory from this period is probably quite vague, though, because your hippocampus only became fully functional once you were around 8 years old.

What you need to know:

- Young children's brains are very busy! They use twice as much energy as yours and most of this energy is being used to build, strengthen and stabilise connections between their brain cells

- When it comes to visualising something that isn't directly there in front of them to help solve a problem, young children's brains are not yet as good as adults'

What to do about this:

- Be careful not to ask young children to draw too heavily on earlier memories while they are problem solving. They can be easily distracted or overwhelmed if they have to do both at once

What else to do

Young children do not have intrinsic awareness of how important a good education is for a successful future! Rather, they are motivated by fun and enjoyment.

A child's sense of its world, together with an ability to move around it, are two of the earliest systems to develop in the brain. This means that interaction and movement should be often recruited when teaching young children. Though few parts of children's brains are usually fully mature, they are primarily limited in their activities by high distractibility and limited capacity for holding things in their mind (working memory again). With this in mind, effective teaching methods could involve the following strategies:

- Teaching through song
- Avoiding too many learning objectives in a single class
- Avoiding heavy reliance on information learnt in previous classes
- Learning through playing games
- Gaining a class's attention at the end of an activity in fun ways

Social junkies – the teenage brain

The good bits

Think back to when you were a teenager…what were you like? Thought you knew better than your parents? Weren't afraid of taking risks and didn't worry about consequences? Did you belong to an inseparable group of friends? These traits don't fit every teenager's experiences but they are quite common and they all have an explanation in the stages of brain development that teenagers experience.

- The teenage brain is close to being fully developed but isn't quite there
- Many parts of the brain are mature, however, and some important long-range connections between different brain areas are in place as well. This enables them to be rather clever and deal with lots of intellectual problems in addition to becoming much more sociable
- Parts of the teenage brain that signal fun and enjoyment, such as the **nucleus accumbens** (the reward bit we mentioned earlier) are also very well developed and these parts play a crucial role in shaping behaviour

Social junkies – the teenage brain

The bad bits

The previous page made the teenager sound jolly, bright and ready to face the big, wide world. However there are some other important things to know:

- The sophisticated **frontal lobe**, which adults use to plan for the future, isn't fully developed in teenagers
- Instead they use the limbic system's primitive **amygdala** to weigh up the appropriateness of emotions
- An important series of connections between **frontal**, **temporal** and **parietal lobes** also remains immature in young teenagers

This means that teenagers can't always put instant gratification and enjoyment in the context of possible future losses, resulting in poor judgment, failure to control impulses and more recklessness (especially when among peers). Remember, too, that teenagers will not always appreciate somebody else's point of view so they need adult guidance, clear social structures and consistent expectations.

Life-long learners – the adult brain

The good bits

As an adult, your brain is sophisticated and mature, capable of highly complex, abstract thoughts and able to create novel and exciting ideas to change the world in which you live. Most important of all, your brain never stops learning! It continues to lay down new memories and, as in childhood, these have their basis in the physical connections between brain cells.

- The greatest ability of your adult brain comes from your fully developed **prefrontal cortex** in your **frontal lobe**
- Your childhood brain was controlled by its **midbrain and limbic system** and was only concerned with enjoyment
- Your teenage brain had some use of its prefrontal cortex but still needed fine-tuning

By adulthood your prefrontal cortex has strong and highly focused connections to beat the primitive impulses and regulate your behaviour to maximise your chances of survival and future success. The prefrontal cortex does this best by identifying whether instant gains are worthwhile in the face of distant losses, and vice versa.

Life-long learners – the adult brain

The not so good bits

It should be pointed out that the way adults learn isn't quite the same as children or teenagers. Adults can clearly still learn new tasks, but some may be easier and quicker to learn than others. Languages, for example, are easier to learn before the age of 7-8 because at this time all phonemes that are regularly being heard are stored in the same language areas in the brain. Subsequently, new phonemes learnt from new languages are stored separately from the native phonemes in the brain and are therefore not as readily accessible.

But staying positive…

… It was once widely believed that certain skills could *only* be learnt before a certain age, in what was termed a **critical period**. That is no longer held to be true. Though it is easier to learn a foreign language as a child, it is not impossible to do so as an adult.

Critical periods are a neuro-myth. Instead we use the term **sensitive period** to indicate that the limits of our learning are not set in stone. We can learn throughout our lives; it may just take a little bit longer to learn some things when we're older.

Future Issues for Brain Science in the Classroom

Cognitive enhancers

Drugs that improve our cognitive performance (eg how well we can concentrate or how much information we can recall) are known as **cognitive enhancers**. Cognitive enhancers are not as new as you might think:

- Cognitive enhancing drugs (eg Ritalin©) have been used for many years in the treatment of ADHD
- They appear to work in a similar way to some drugs of abuse – amphetamine is used as a cognitive enhancer
- They increase the amount of **dopamine** in the brain, in the gaps between neurons

Although this makes them sound dangerous, the fact is we really don't know what their long-term effects are. At present they are most commonly used by university students and are illegal when used in this way. However, this is definitely an area of neuroscience on the move – so watch this space!

Where do you draw the line?

Many of us would argue that society benefits by having people with psychiatric and learning disabilities.

Some disorders, including **dyslexia**, may be accompanied by specific benefits. It is no secret, for example, that Albert Einstein was dyslexic.

In the case of **bipolar disorder** – which involves the emotional cycling between manic, highly creative periods and highly depressive periods, and has been associated with some famous artists – many people who are on medication to control the swings of mood greatly miss the creative periods they once had. Think about it, if medication had been available at the time would you have prescribed it to Van Gogh?

Such questions are becoming increasingly relevant as drug technologies develop.

Hypnosis and learning?

Hypnosis is not just a wacky parlour trick, as may appear to be the case when you watch a TV hypnosis show. Cognitive neuroscience has increased our understanding of how hypnosis affects brain function.

This has led some neuroscientists, notably Sarah-Jayne Blakemore and Uta Frith*, to suggest that it may be possible to use hypnosis and associated deep relaxation to enhance learning. However, the effects of such approaches would probably vary according to how hypnotisable the subjects were. There is a normal distribution of hypnotic susceptibility: about 15% of people are highly susceptible to hypnotic suggestions.

This, of course, raises ethical issues similar to those in stage hypnosis. However, although there is still some disagreement about the potential dangers of hypnosis, there is a general consensus about its benefits when used correctly.

See page 125

Brain-machine interfaces

Imagine a world in which you could surf the internet merely by thinking about it – a world in which you could directly communicate with another person without the need to utter a single sound. Sounds impossible, doesn't it? Not necessarily.

- Research carried out to try and allow amputees and people with spinal cord injuries to be able to move artificial limbs by thought alone has given scientists a wealth of information about the hidden language of the brain – the crackle and fizz of electro-chemical communication among brain cells
- Although scientists still have a great deal to learn about how the brain stores information, not to mention how it generates thought and movement, it might be possible one day to use machines to augment brain performance

If this were possible the real question would be would you want it? Perhaps one day such interfaces will be perceived no differently than taking a calculator into a maths exam is today.

Neuro-education

The greatest future issue, in many ways, is brain science in the classroom itself. At the heart of this are two key areas:

- Ensuring that scientifically acquired knowledge is described accurately and is not distorted so that learners do not acquire misinformation about the brain. (After all, we would not find it acceptable to teach children that Henry VIII had 9 wives)
- Making sure we do not lose effective teacher practice that is not wrong in itself but has been poorly described using brain science terminology (like being 'left or right brained')

To achieve this, teachers and neuroscientists will need to:
- Communicate with each other and see each other at work in their native environments (from classroom to laboratory)
- Be aware of and have respect for the different language they speak, the very different research methods they use and what these different methods can and cannot tell us

Reflective Summary

So what does brain science actually say?

In many ways neuroscience doesn't contradict what we know about the processes of effective learning from a social point of view. In fact, much of it concretises effective good practice in teaching by emphasising the key things that all good teachers know:

- Keep learning interesting and stimulating and use repetition in clever ways so that your learners' brains are constantly required to be actively engaged
- Teach children to have a positive mindset about their potential as learners – and share the brain science that demonstrates this
- Be nice to your students' brains by maintaining a positive emotional climate – they will learn more in the end

And to be blunt, if you do a lot of repetition the same way without much engagement you will be less effective. If you do whizzy, engaging lessons with no repetition you will also be less effective. You need both, not just to maintain motivation but also to ensure effective brain function generally.

Review

Introduction

- Learning happens in the brain and the brain changes in response to external environment and to experiences

- Only about a third of brain connections associated with intelligence form automatically in early childhood as a result of genetics. The rest are the result of the environment a child grows up in

- Teaching children about the brain can help them to become better learners

- It's really interesting stuff!

Brain Bits

- Experience and learning are a balancing act between the different parts of the brain: the hindbrain (or reptilian brain); the midbrain and limbic system – responsible for drives and desires; and the forebrain – the thinking bit

- However, remember that the whole brain is working all the time and every part of the brain is active in every situation. Dividing the brain into bits is just a useful anatomical description based on what things look like

- There are lots of fun ways to teach children about the brain with potential benefits

Review

 The Learning Process

- Learning involves the excitation of neurons – literally

- It is interconnectivity that enables intelligence – therefore experience counts most

- In terms of retention and memory the key is to carefully balance and make use of the **salience** (novelty and relevance) of the information and **repetition**

- Create a web of interconnectivity and association in your teaching that parallels the processes that take place in the creation of long-term memory

- The more you learn the better you get at learning

 The Neuroscience of Memory

- Attention is fundamental to the process of memory – if you don't grab attention then the brain can be very unimpressed

- Emotions and mood also affect learning so also pay attention to these

- Be aware of the different types of attention and the implications for the classroom

- Just because information has entered working memory doesn't mean that it will enter long-term memory – what you do as a teacher matters

- Chunking is a great way to enhance memory

Review

 In the Classroom

- Be aware of what can go wrong with memory and have strategies to deal with it

- Structure lessons to ensure a significant number of high retention points (striking visual imagery, repetition, association, memory and shorter learning episodes joined together)

- When it comes to memory we are all highly visual at a certain level – make use of this in the classroom. Recognise the importance of using a continuous schedule of positive reward to release dopamine (catch the children doing the right thing and they will do it again). Use humour

- Use modelling (the demonstration of skills) to enhance learning and give mirror neurons what they want

 The Developing Brain

- Young brains are busy but aren't good at visualising something that isn't there whilst solving problems. When students are problem solving, don't ask them to draw too heavily on earlier memories

- The teenage brain is a bright social junkie but needs clear guidance and boundaries

- Although some things may be harder to learn with age we can all learn at any time

- Critical periods are a neuro-myth, so be careful how you think about potential at different ages

Review

 Future Issues for Brain Science in the Classroom

- Drugs can improve cognitive performance. How we control this may be an issue
- Just because one day we might be able to interfere with brain structure, should we?
- Brain-machine interfacing may one day be possible
- Neuroscience and education are different fields of study and still have a long way to go in talking to each other

Finally, some top tips for taking this learning forward as a reflective practitioner:

- You don't need to speak the language of neuroscience to improve memory and retention using the basic principles
- Take an action learning approach to implementing changes (test it out, see how it works and modify your practice when you have seen an impact)

Recommended reading

If you'd like to learn more about brain structures and scientific terminology in a fun way, download the fabulous iPod App *3D Brain*, produced by Dolan DANA Learning Centre at Cold Spring Harbor Lab. 2010 (wish we had come up with this!)

To find out more about the neuroscience of learning by two neuroscientists read: *The Learning Brain: Lessons for Education* by Sarah-Jayne Blakemore and Uta Frith. Blackwell Publishing, 2005

Or read more about the issues and debates in this area in: *Neuroscience and Education: Issues and Opportunities*, by the Teaching and Learning Research Programme and the Economic and Social Research Council, 2007

For a general introduction about the brain with some great pictures see: *The Brain Book* by Rita Carter. Dorling Kindersley, 2009

Take your understanding even further by reading: *The Private Life of the Brain* by Susan Greenfield, Penguin Books, 2000

For a couple of perspectives on learning and brain science from two academics with education backgrounds you might also like to read: *Introducing Neuroeducational Research: neuroscience, education and the brain from contexts to practice* by Paul Howard-Jones, Routledge, 2010

The Brain at School: Educational Neuroscience in the Classroom by John Geake, Open University Press, 2009.

About the authors

Eleanor Dommett

Eleanor is a Lecturer in Biological Psychology at the Open University and has previously held positions at Oxford University, Somerville College and Lady Margaret Hall where she has conducted research and teaching in a variety of different areas of neuroscience. She has also been involved in large scale neuroeducation research, supported by the CfBT and led by the Institute for the Future of the Mind at Oxford University. In her own laboratory at the Open University she focuses on the mechanisms of action of drugs such as amphetamine and methylphenidate, both of which are used in the treatment of ADHD as well as for cognitive enhancement in healthy individuals. In addition to her research she continues to contribute to a variety of areas of teaching, most recently writing and editing material on sensory neuroscience. She is passionate about raising public understanding of science and to this end contributes articles to the Times Education Supplement, Science in Parliament magazine and frequently visits schools to work with both pupils and teachers. She is also recorder for the Education Section of the British Science Festival. ellie.dommett@open.ac.uk

About the authors

Ian Devonshire

Ian is a Research Fellow in the School of Life Sciences at the University of Nottingham and has previously held positions at the Universities of Oxford and Sheffield. He became interested in the workings of the human brain at a young age and enrolled on one of the very first Neuroscience degree courses offered in the UK. His laboratory research currently focuses on how the developing brain can be changed by its environment but he also conducts classroom-based research to find the most fun and effective forms of science outreach. To this end, Ian regularly visits schools and colleges with a suitcase full of brains! ian.devonshire@nottingham.ac.uk

Richard Churches

Richard is Principal Adviser for Research and Evidence Based Practice at CfBT Education Trust, the world-leading education consultancy, charity and investor in research. He was an Advanced Skills Teacher and senior manager in challenging inner city schools and has taught in a top grammar school, international school and a special school (MLD). As well as being a writer, researcher and government adviser, he has worked as a teacher, trainer and consultant in the UK and overseas, including: Abu Dhabi, Bahrain, Dubai, the Netherlands, the Irish Republic, India, Italy, Jordan, Kuwait, Oman, Pakistan, Qatar, South Africa, US. He is a doctoral researcher at the University of Surrey where he is investigating the relationship between charismatic leadership oratory, hypnosis and altered state of consciousness. r.churches@surrey.ac.uk

Order form

Your details

Name _____

Position _____

School _____

Address _____

_____

_____

Telephone _____

Fax _____

E-mail _____

VAT No. (EC only) _____

Your Order Ref _____

Please send me:

No. copies

Learning & The Brain _____ Pocketbook [ ]

_____ Pocketbook [ ]

_____ Pocketbook [ ]

_____ Pocketbook [ ]

Order by Post
Teachers' Pocketbooks
Laurel House, Station Approach
Alresford, Hants. SO24 9JH UK

Order by Phone, Fax or Internet
Telephone: +44 (0)1962 735573
Facsimile: +44 (0)1962 733637
E-mail: sales@teacherspocketbooks.co.uk
Web: www.teacherspocketbooks.co.uk

Customers in USA should contact:
2427 Bond Street, University Park, IL 60466
Tel: 866 620 6944   Facsimile: 708 534 7803
E-mail: mp.orders@ware-pak.com
Web: www.managementpocketbooks.com